Contents

The purpose of this book...........................

Physical 5

Social 9

Financial...18

Sexual 24

Emotional 33

Self-esteem...38

Children (AKA: attempting to co-parent with a controller)...........43

What helped others survive and escape 54

Strategies for dealing with difficult people 57

Breaking Free: Recognising & Surviving Controlling Behaviours

By Eva Jean (Copyright 2021)

The purpose of this book

I want this book to save lives. Not just helping one more woman escape a controller before she is badly harmed or worse, but to save a woman **time**, helping them reclaim their happiness and freedom and their life back.

The purpose of this book is to help readers recognise themselves in the situations shown.

I also want to show that even allowing for the fact that every situation is unique, and every controller and survivor individual, we must never forget this fact: **control is control**.

No matter how soundly it is justified, or how bad we feel about ourselves, **control is control**. Control can be extremely dangerous, and it usually escalates in severity.

I did originally try to pack a lot more into this book. In doing so, the goal became complicated, because my original aim was to **catalogue controlling behaviours, for the purpose of helping those feeling trapped by them.** That was it.

Maybe that book is for another day, or another person. But for now, I want to keep this information simple, and easy to access. This book is a catalogue of controlling behaviours, divided into areas, with a foreword providing a little context on each.

I have divided the areas of control into the following sections: **physical, social, financial, sexual, emotional, self-esteem, children** *(shared parenting with a controller)*.

I wanted to detail as much as possible, because there are as many deviations in controlling behaviours as there are people on the planet; two different people carrying out violence may do so in very different ways. One controller may use physical force very readily; another may only have to whisper something in your ear to have you shaking from fear.

I have also included chapters with official advice for if you want to escape a relationship, details of what has helped others survive and escape, as well as strategies for dealing for difficult people **if you have no choice** i.e. your abusive ex who is also the father of your child, a family member you have to see occasionally, or a work colleague.

DISCLAIMER: For the sake of continuity and simplicity I have addressed survivors as female and controllers as male. Obviously, this is not always the case. In terms of official domestic violence figures, most survivors or victims are female. However, ANYBODY can be helped by this book, male or female, whatever your sexuality – if you are trying to **break free**, I support you wholeheartedly.

You can email me at evajeanwriter@gmail.com

Let's **break free.** We all deserve happiness.

EVA XXX

Areas of control:

Physical

A bit about physical control

Physical forms of control don't just involve physical violence or assault; they can be present in many other more subtle forms.

Physical violence doesn't necessarily mean a person is bigger and stronger than you; your controller may be physically smaller than you, but still using physical control. This is all about power. It is all about the *threat* of someone using their body or their physicality in some way to get you to **do** something, or to **stop you** from doing something.

By the same token, someone who is using violence may seem 'meek' to others, which can mean you feel an extra struggle to confide in anyone, because it may not seem feasible that you are being attacked, or threatened, or intimidated. Somebody can be menacing without using physical force, but they can also use their greater size to intimidate you. It is worth remembering that physical violence is *never* okay in a relationship. It is also worth realising that it is extremely common, if not expected, that a controlling and abusive partner will likely have **two distinct sides** to his personality; a face he wears out in **public**, and a face he presents to you **behind closed doors. He hides this side for a reason.**

My father was absolutely terrifying without laying a hand on any of us. He was menacing with a glare, a growl, a spiteful remark, body-blocking, and once, when I began to argue back, the raising of a fist.

He was menacing just by walking into a room, and everyone used to scarper.

When he was upset, he would drink a bottle of wine, and his behaviour would change further. We would all hide. My mother told me recently that she used to barricade the bedroom door to keep him out.

Here are some examples of physical control (bear in mind that there will be some overlap between areas of control, and you may see some of these examples crop up again in other areas):

Your controller scaring you

Preventing you from leaving a room or area

Using their body to block you or stop you or intimidate you – 'body-blocking'

Behaving in a menacing manner

Sulking because you won't give in (this may seem harmless, and we all probably do it at times, but a pathological controller will sulk to such effect and extent, that it has an almost physical effect on you, on the room, on others)

Dominating a room or environment

Causing discomfort in other people

Being a 'mood hoover'

Intimidating or being abusive or unkind to you or your friends/family

Shouting at you

Carrying out ANY intended physical harm against you

Being aggressive or passive/aggressive

Mocking you

Invading your personal space in a way that is threatening or unwanted

Kicking you

Grabbing you

Shoving you

Strangling you

Pinching you

Causing you to fear for your life

Hitting, punching, or slapping you

Using tools or items to inflict pain or punishment on you when it is unwarranted and unwanted

Using physical punishment when you disagree with them

Using physical punishment when you go against their wishes

Using their body to hold or weigh you down

Using force during sex that is unwarranted or unwanted

Using force to rape or assault you

Using force or threats to force you to carry out sexual acts

Ordering you about

Frightening you and forcing you to do things

Glaring

Growling

Refusing to move

Refusing to let you leave the house

Locking the doors and windows

Taking your keys and refusing to give them back

Refusing to let you wash or take care of yourself

Breaking or smashing things to frighten you

Breaking or smashing things to prevent you from using them

Smashing things to frighten you

Laughing in your face in order to humiliate and intimidate

Ignoring you as a form of control or humiliation

Spitting at you

Drinking alcohol and behaving aggressively

Taking drugs and behaving aggressively

Using alcohol or drugs to excuse violence

Inflicting bruises on you and forcing you to hide them

Denying you medical attention when it is needed, i.e. hiding your phone, refusing to call 999, trying to stop you seeing your doctor, hiding your medication

Engaging in ANY physical activity towards you that is unwanted and is causing you distress

Forcing you to over-eat

Force-feeding you

Drugging you

Forcing you to take drugs that sedate you

Restraining or tying you up

This list is not exhaustive.

Areas of control:

Social

A bit about social control

A relationship that involves somebody limiting your social network and isolating you from friends, family, social groups, interests – no matter how gradually it is done – is **never healthy** - and is a common control tactic. I don't think I have heard, read about, or experienced a controlling relationship where this didn't happen in some form.

We could become isolated because of the controller putting pressure on us to not see people, or creating such drama that whenever we *do* actually get out or talk to people, we are exhausted, tainted by the guilt we have been manipulated into feeling, and, over time, simply stop trying to socialise because of the hassle and the fallout. If we let them, controllers can taint every positive thing we have to look forward to. They gradually destroy our support network bit by bit.

Being isolated from outside influences (any influences outside of the controller) is surprisingly effective. When we lack social support, we lose perspective and that 'sounding board' and emotional support that we all need. There is no doubt that the controller will feel extremely threatened by your friendships, or in fact anything you enjoy that makes you feel good. **This is because they want you unhappy, and not distracted by anything that stops them from having your full attention at all times.**

The more isolated you are, the less support you have and the lower your self-worth, your self-esteem. The lower you feel, the more vulnerable you are to the controller's manipulations and bashes to your confidence. In time you may even begin to feel that you don't deserve anything more than toxicity.

There is a further element to isolation; having you all to themselves. They keep ultimate control over their main source of ego-boost: **you**. Keeping you by their side as much as possible. A further element can be making you account for your every move and action, so that you are too afraid to even try and be your own person and make new friends. Social control is a vicious cycle, because once they have achieved their goal, it is hard to break out of that supreme isolation once all the cogs of the control 'machine' are operating and you are completely trapped, contained, with nobody to talk to and nothing to look forward to.

The fewer people there are around you, the fewer people the controller has to attempt to charm or manipulate. If someone is a compulsive liar, this means less lies being told to less people.

The controller wants you to believe that they are the only source of information and attention worth having. By allowing yourself to become isolated, you prove their point; that you are inferior to them, that you need them and nobody else. **Put simply, the weaker you are, the less you'll fight.**

Sometimes control ramps up if you have a baby together. This is very common, and according to domestic violence statistics, many relationships turn increasingly controlling once a baby is born. A turning point for me came after my daughter was born:

> *When my daughter was a few months old, I wanted to volunteer a couple of afternoons a week at a local charity shop. I had given up my full-time job to care for her, and the then-controller was working full time. His grandmother lived a few minutes away and was happy to look after her. He absolutely did not want me volunteering. We fought bitterly for days, and he made me feel terrible about having depression and needing to have a break and get out of the house a few hours a week. One of his accusations was: 'I thought you **wanted** to have a baby?' I never forgot those words and the guilt they created.*
>
> *When I didn't back down, the controller then insisted on applying to volunteer with me, so that 'we could be together.' When I went quiet, he got moody, and stated that I had 'made it clear I didn't want him to do this.' I reasoned that I wasn't trying to hurt him or my family, that I had always worked and been out of the house and was missing the social aspects of work. I fought my corner, and I applied to volunteer at a charity shop I loved, two afternoons a week. I volunteered there for a year, making many friends. It was the right decision for me, and it really gave me a boost, helping me*

through my low mood. It made me begin to feel like 'me' again, and he was very threatened by this. I think because he couldn't (or wouldn't) physically stop me from doing what I needed to do, he appeared to back down. However, he continued to punish me for leaving the house by taking our daughter and going to his grandmother's. He never told me that he would do this.

I told him of my start and finish times, so that he would know when I was back home. However, he would conveniently 'forget' this, and every time I finished my shift, I would get home just after 5pm to an empty, dark and messy house. He was punishing me for needing something for myself, and I remember feeling like I wasn't part of a family anymore.

A common contradiction is a controller demanding of you what they will not themselves give. I was expected to be at home and wait on him. Yet whenever he left the house, when I asked where he was going, he would reply, 'Out.' If I asked roughly when he would be back, he would say 'I'm back when I'm back.' He treated my question with contempt.

Another example of social control:

I was having my first night out locally with an old friend. My friend came a long way to see me, and we planned my first night out since having my daughter. The controller seemed okay with it at first, but grew increasingly sulky, quizzing me as to why I needed to go out and 'leave him and our baby.'

I said he was welcome to come, but as he 'hated dance music and dancing,' he refused.

Considering I had left my job, been looking after our baby almost 24/7, and had suffered postnatal depression, this was a bit of a welcome change of scene for me, and previously, I had enjoyed regular nights out. In fact, the controller had previously said he liked this about me; that I was outgoing and fun loving. The two of us had gone out drinking together when we first dated, and now, a year or so later, he was like a different person, sullen, argumentative, and not wanting to leave the house except for work.

My friend and I listened to music and enjoyed getting ready together. The controller sulked the whole time and was quite rude to my friend.

He told me he didn't like what I was wearing (a long skirt and a nice top). The final control tactic was him trying to 'pin me down' to a time I would be returning home. I said I didn't know, but it would be by around 3am, as I liked a dance, and a few drinks. He knew not to worry about me, and that my friends and I would look out for each other. He then said that he would refuse to go to bed until I was home, and that he would sit up and wait for me. I was so incredibly exasperated by this point, telling him there was no point!

When I got back home (the town centre was a ten-minute walk from town) having had a great time, the controller was indeed sitting up, with a face like thunder. I remember feeling like he was my father, miserable and oppressive, despite him being so much younger than me. At that moment I remember realising who I truly was, despite his constant attempts to crush my spirit. I was fun loving, and a loyal friend, a good mother, a loving partner. He was insecure, controlling, and immune to reason.

Examples of social control:

The controller wanting you to be with them all the time

The controller getting upset when your phone rings or you get a message

The controller getting upset when you talk to anyone else, even long-term friends or family

Them checking your phone, reading your messages

Them deleting messages from your friends, denying that you received any

Making you show them texts

Questioning why you have certain contacts on your phone

Demanding control of your phone i.e. 'holding it for you, because you cannot be trusted'

Making you justify every friendship

Using your friends/family/hobbies/work to query why they, the controller, are *'not enough for you'*

Not wanting you to speak to a doctor or medical professional, when you need help

Belittling medical professionals

Threatening to end the relationship if you seek medical help

Refusing to come with you, or refusing to take you to an appointment

Them coming to the appointment, but talking for you, or being 'overbearing'

Claiming that they have all the medical knowledge you need

Not wanting you to take medication that could help you

An example of medical/social control: after my baby was born, I developed postnatal depression; it was severe, and I was overwhelmed and struggling to bond. It was a traumatic birth. I cried a lot, and when I talked to the controller about needing to go and see my doctor because something was very wrong, he responded with annoyance. He told me I 'shouldn't need to go and see a doctor, as it felt like a threat to him as he should be able to fix me.' When I made an appointment, he insisted on coming with me.

*My doctor was very kind and compassionate, and when she asked me how I was, the controller proceeded to talk over me and answer for me. I realised how insane and irrational this was: after denying that I needed medical help, the controller was now explaining **my** feelings to the very doctor he had wanted to stop me from seeing. Thankfully, I was prescribed medication to help, and was encouraged to see that lovely doctor several times on my own, as I recovered. Interestingly she commented on how controlling he had seemed.*

Not allowing you to have a social media profile

Insisting that they have all your passwords/login details

Insisting on a shared profile when there is no need for this

Insisting on a shared profile so that they can monitor your conversations and friends

Not allowing you any privacy

Quizzing your friends or work colleagues about you

Stalking you at work, even if you have split up

Trying to get close to old work colleagues or friends after you have split up

Wanting to be with you every second of every day

Them sulking, guilt-tripping you when you want to go out, or have arranged a plan with someone

Turning up to personal activities such as a 'girly get-together' under the guise of 'just passing by'

Checking up on you

Questioning your social plans

Texting or calling you constantly, in order to stop you relaxing with friends

Accusing your friends of being controlling (this is 'projection,' where a controller projects their own negative behaviour onto somebody else)

Commenting that certain friends are a 'bad influence' on you, or that you tend to 'act out' when around certain people

Attending social events with you, but then sabotaging them by sulking, refusing to socialise, or punishing you afterwards

Feeling threatened by you having fun at social events

Insisting on you staying by their side constantly

Shadowing you

Butting in on conversations you are having with others

Having to account for every move

Being accused of cheating if you talk to another person

Being accused of cheating if you WANT to talk to anyone else

Being accused of cheating if you want some freedom or independence

Not allowing you any freedom to make decisions

Not wanting you to make social decisions or make friends or connections, *especially if this is a very strong part of your personality*

Stopping you from looking nice or dressing up

Being/acting insecure around opposite sex friendships (for example) for no good reason

Implying that every man you talk to wants to sleep with you

Behaving aggressively with others in public

Walking with his hand on the back of your neck (this can be a controlling action)

Belittling your friendships in subtle or overt ways

Trying to turn friends against you by telling lies to you/your friends *(be aware that a pathological liar is likely lying to everyone they speak to, not just you; everyone gets a different version of the truth)*

Questioning your 'loyalty to the relationship' every time you try to socialise, or a friend contacts you

Being possessive over your time

Making schedules for your time

Being overbearing

Creating a drama just before you are due to leave the house

Belittling or undermining you, so that you don't feel confident enough to socialise

Insisting that you don't need anyone

Insisting that your family are no good (when in fact they lift you up)

Mocking and embarrassing you in front of friends

Acting sullen whilst out socialising, so that you feel pressured to come home

Causing fights with your friends

Examples of more extreme social control could include:

Tracking your car or phone

Hiring a Private Detective to follow you

Following you around, turning up to places you are at **(stalking is known to be a high-risk behaviour in controlling relationships, and can be a precursor to violence)**

Installing hidden cameras (a **gross** invasion of privacy, and in fact illegal)

Using the police to 'rein you in' – an example of this: an older controller I was with for many years, was insecure and jealous because of my friendships. The relationship was deteriorating rapidly. I had a night out planned with friends. I told the controller about it and told him that I would be packing an overnight bag and staying with a friend as we would be out late, and the last train left early.

The controller was not in the habit of texting much, but that night whilst I was out sitting in a bar with friends, he messaged me constantly, making his unhappiness towards me clear. I believe he was trying to keep my attention on him and spoil my night. The night before, we had argued; he had tried to dissuade me from going out, but I was feeling smothered and said I was going. That tactic hadn't worked, so now the constant texting and upsetting me began. The messages became increasingly aggressive and frightening, with him using **CAPITALS TO INTIMIDATE.** *He told me that I was not 'behaving like a wife,' and that 'I would need to make the decision to put him above my social life,' or similar. This was extremely distressing; his messages felt threatening. I eventually became so upset that he was ruining a night I had been looking forward to for days, I switched off my phone. He knew of my plans, that I was safe, and that I would be back home the next day. I was sick of him being domineering, and I told him so.*

Later that night at my friend's house, I turned my phone back on to find missed calls and a voicemail left by the police.

The controller had, in a rage, called the police and reported me missing. He had lied and told them that I wasn't answering my phone, and that he was 'concerned for my safety' because I had not 'checked in with him.' In a final act of control and humiliation, he told the police that he had no idea as to my whereabouts, so that the police were forcing me to report in person to the local station, so that they could confirm I was safe. To say I was livid, and that the relationship was completely dead for me at that point, is an understatement. I believe his actions were a punishment, and his purpose was to force me to 'toe the line' and behave in the way he expected me to behave.

Do not underestimate how far a controller will go to dominate you if they feel that you are not behaving in the way they want you to behave. Controlling behaviours tend to escalate. Several women are killed intentionally every week in the UK alone because of domestic violence.

Areas of control:

Financial

A bit about financial control

Finances, and using money to control, is quite a common area of domestic abuse. Many times, it can be overlooked, as the controller may convince us that what they are doing is what is 'best for us' and that we 'cannot be trusted' to run our own lives. They may also use 'traditional' frameworks to bully us into conforming to what may have been considered 'normal' fifty or sixty years ago, before women had equal rights regarding earning their own money, working, and having independence if they wanted it.

Financial control could include the withholding of money, the allocation of money, as well as overseeing every financial decision we make, or forcing us to justify our spending. It can also include forcing us to spend excessive amounts on the controller, or getting into debt **(don't forget, the controller needs us unhealthy and unhappy so that control is easier.)**

Here are some examples of financial control:

Your controller insisting on managing all the finances

Shutting you down whenever you try to discuss this

Forcing you to pay your wages into their account, or an account that only they can access

Having housekeeping meted out to you in tiny dribs and drabs because you 'cannot be trusted'

Being told you are not capable of making financial decisions

Having your intelligence questioned or insulted

Having to beg or 'barter' for the money you need

Having to justify essentials like food or toilet roll

Being forced to re-use tissues or ration food to an excessive degree

Refusing to let you go shopping without them

Following you when you shop

'Shadowing' your every move

Timing you when you leave the house

Starting arguments or questioning why you need to go grocery shopping

Being accused of cheating on them every time you leave the house

Checking money excessively and counting the change you bring back

Hiding bank cards from you

Keeping your bank card because you 'cannot be trusted'

Changing PIN numbers without telling you, to make you feel or look stupid

Refusing to give you login details

Them being secretive with their own money and spending

Forcing you to show them all the shopping you bought

Getting angry or aggressive with you when you buy something that cheers you up, that they haven't 'authorised' like a magazine or bar of chocolate

Accusing you of stealing money or having sex with strangers for money

Them having resentment towards you because you earn more

Having resentment towards you making your own decisions with your money

Having resentment that you work or are self-employed

Getting irritable and trying to 'bring you down off your high horse' because you are excited about something you bought

Ignoring you when you try to show them something pleasing

Them lying about money

Them making bad decisions or frittering money away, whilst accusing you of doing the same thing (this is called 'projection')

Implying that he has more money than he does

Lying about the work he does (this can indicate a pathological liar)

Lying to you about how much money you have jointly

Lying to your family about how much money there is

Asking your family to lie to you about money

I want to give an example of a controlling partner lying about money and asking your family to lie to you, because it happened to me, and it was one of the first major red flags that something was very wrong, and that I was systematically being lied to about small and large things.

We'd had our baby, who was premature, and I was living in the hospital with her, quite poorly myself. The controller was promising me that we had plenty of money and that he was taking care of everything back at home financially and house-wise. I was obviously extremely vulnerable at the time, and had to trust him, because I couldn't physically leave the hospital and did not have transport.

When I finally checked our bank balance at the cashpoint in the hospital, there was a much lower amount than he was claiming there was. Hundreds of pounds less. This obviously caused me huge stress on top of all the other worries. When I confronted him about why he had lied, he was not concerned about my feelings or perspective. He was only concerned that he needed me to trust him and believe him when he told me things. So rather than feeling remorse at his end, there was only anger and irritation that I didn't take his word as gospel. He later claimed that he lied to protect me.

It also transpired previously that he had asked my mother and my sister to lie to me about how much a particular item cost. He wanted them to 'back up' his lie. They thankfully refused, and my mother came and gently spoke to me about it, as it obviously concerned her that the father of my child was lying to me. Interestingly, when I confronted him about why he would lie to me and ask my family to lie, he denied it had happened, insisting that my family were 'telling me what I wanted to hear.'

I remember feeling frustrated, and responding with, 'But why would I ever want to hear that you are lying to me and asking my family to lie too?' He didn't have an answer to that. He sulked and refused to address the issue.

When things just do not feel right, and you cannot put your finger on why, trust your gut. Dig a little deeper. Your instincts are there to protect you.

More examples of financial control:

Them spending money on frivolous things or things you didn't want, and then using this to manipulate you by calling you 'ungrateful' or 'boring'

Bragging or lying about how much they 'spoil' you or spend on you, when actually they are doing no such thing

Giving away money but denying you any

Being more giving with their friends or your friends than they are with you (this can send you the message that you are not as important to them as other people)

Repeatedly gambling away or 'losing' money that you need, and then insisting that it is your fault

Constantly asking you for money, and denying it happened (this is **GASLIGHTING**)

Them acting like an authority on finances

Them insulting or devaluing you because you wish to seek outside/professional advice

Them devaluing professional financial services

Them making it clear that you should only talk to THEM, not anybody else

Them getting angry or threatened because you have done your own research

Being forced or coerced into buying expensive items for the controller, especially items that are completely unnecessary but related to 'status' in their eyes, such as designer trainers

Being forced or coerced into taking out loans in their name, because they have bad credit, or bad spending habits, or just for the hell of it

I have seen this happen to several people, with devastating, far-reaching effects. I want to talk about this because nobody thinks it will happen to them, especially if you currently have trust in the person and relationship.

It is very easy to underestimate how far a controller will go to keep control over you, especially if the relationship ends. I call this 'revenge control' because it has the capacity to cause hurt and pain, and possibly severe debt problems for many years.

In one instance the victim had been persuaded to take out a ten-thousand-pound loan in her name, because her then partner was reckless with spending, and wanted to splash out on gadgets and cars. He of course promised to pay her back the money, but then when the relationship ended shortly after, he attempted to keep control by refusing to pay off the outstanding debt. Because the debt was in her name, there wasn't a thing she could do. She lost her flat because she couldn't afford to pay the rent, and she had to move back in with family and take out an IVA (Individual Voluntary Arrangement). She is hoping to get a mortgage in the future, but possibly cannot because of this debt. She now has very little money for herself. Because of her ex's immaturity and selfish need to control, she may have lost that dream for her future.

*

In another instance, a victim was persuaded to pay for her partner's mobile phone contract. Again, the details were all in her name. He ran up high bills and she, not earning much above minimum wage as it was, was legally obligated to pay for his recklessness without any care for her feelings, nor any remorse. When she finally left him, he ramped up his control, insisting that she met up with him privately so that he could pay back the debt. When she began dating again, her ex used these meetings to criticise her new boyfriend, belittling him. She eventually had to start asserting herself, insisting that he stop his behaviour, because her new relationship was nothing to do with him.

By giving into her ex's demands and even interacting with him at all, she was still allowing him power over her. When she stopped meeting up with her ex, and blocked

him on social media, he lost his power over her. She was able to move forward and allow her loving new relationship to thrive.

More examples:

Being told that your money is not your own to manage

The controller telling other people that you can't manage money

Feeling pressured to spend or shop in ways that aren't comfortable to you

Being made to do 'demeaning' things in order to be given money

The controller not paying their way

(After you have separated) The controller refusing to pay towards housing costs (if you share a mortgage), or their child

Areas of control...

Sexual

Funny how sexual control is the hardest area to write about and think about. Therefore, it's likely to be the hardest area to read about. Do yourself a favour – be kind to yourself. If you are struggling to read these examples, especially if they are bringing up some kind of trauma, take regular breaks. Drink tea, talk to a friend, watch a happy film. Break it up and do it in stages.

I did try to figure out why sexual control was so hard to write about. It's because of the **shame** involved. We seem to have shame attached to our sexuality more so than any other area of control. And if we have been exploited, or treated badly, manipulated into believing it is all our fault – the shame we will have been made to feel can be tenfold.

Let's begin with some examples:

The controller fetishizing you / denying your worth as a whole person

The controller watching excessive porn in front of you and comparing you to the models

Watching excessive porn and then coercing you into 'acting out' scenarios they like

Denying you sex

Having affairs and telling you it is your fault

Having affairs and blaming your looks or personality

Rejecting affection or intimacy with you

Controlling how you have sex

Making sex all about 'them' and what they like

*

Threatening rape

Raping you, then telling you it was your fault

Enforcing sex i.e. "you need to do your duty,"

Guilt-tripping you if you don't feel like it, or are tired

Wearing you down until you give in (this can happen in a long-term relationship, or on a date. 'Date rape' is still rape)

I experienced a date like this, with a man who bragged constantly, and was very pushy. He was physically small, and I didn't feel threatened. He talked about his ex and how she didn't deserve him, how she wouldn't give him sex. I was tired and had been working for hours on my laptop. We talked lots. He barely gave me a minute to think. He brought over two bottles of wine, and proceeded to keep topping up my glass. I hadn't eaten much, and eventually I was pretty drunk. When I tried to get into my kitchen to get food, he kept insisting on a kiss. He was stood blocking the kitchen.

We ended up in bed, because he wouldn't take no for an answer. During sex I had a sudden and extreme sensation of 'leaving my body,' – looking at myself, saying, 'What the hell are you doing?' I burst into tears and told him I didn't want to be doing this. I remember curling up on my side, exhausted, just crying. He seemed very uncomfortable, but he wouldn't leave. He was behaving very strangely. He stayed and he wouldn't shut up. He was acting as if nothing had happened. I didn't know it at the time, but I was in shock; I was curled up on the sofa, staring into space. I wanted him to go away so that I could process what had just happened.

When he left, I locked the door, and rang a close friend, who asked me, 'Do you feel like you have been raped?' I burst into tears because it was exactly how I felt. I was grateful that he had said it, rather than me.

I boil washed my sheets that night. It took me a few days to stop feeling angry and tearful. I realised he had come to my house with one intention only – to have sex. And even my tiredness, hesitation, and distress, hadn't put him off from continuing with his tactics until I gave in.

Be aware of controlling behaviours on dates; it shows a distinct lack of boundaries and empathy. If a controller is controlling on a first date, what will they be like in the future?

Further examples:

Body blocking you

Touching you inappropriately when you have already said no

Following you, shadowing you

Making you uncomfortable in any way

Getting angry when you have said no

Sulking

Giving you the silent treatment because you don't want sex

Wheedling or begging you for sex, trying to appeal to your sense of pity

Ignoring boundaries

Getting in your face

Sexually harassing you in **ANY** way – face to face, by phone, text, or on social media

*

Using sex as a punishment, as a way to hurt you

Using sex to be violent towards you

Using sex to humiliate you or make you feel demeaned

Convincing or making you watch adult content you are not comfortable with

Persuading you to make porn, so that you feel 'worthy' or 'desirable'

Convincing you to make sexual photos or videos, then threatening you (even jokingly) with making them public **(doing this is a crime, and is known as 'revenge porn' – it is commonly threatened after a relationship has ended)**

Insulting your appearance

Making you feel ugly or worthless

Comparing you unfavourably to women in the street or on the television, i.e. "Why can't you look more like her?" "If you were as slim as her, I would fancy you more." **Not only is this downright rude and disrespectful, it's abusive.**

Making lewd comments in front of you

Making lewd comments about you, in front of or to others (this is humiliation)

Bragging about you to others

Calling you a slut or a slag

Talking about past sexual conquests to make you feel insecure

Mentioning **your** past conquests to attempt to shame you

Threatening to leave if you don't give him what he wants

Telling you that nobody else will want you

Bragging about affairs to you

*

Expecting a certain level of sex all of the time, regardless of your feelings or needs

Demanding sex **especially** after you have argued or fallen out (this can be a way to regain control)

Demanding sex because they know it makes you tired

Demanding sex to try and stop you leaving

Demanding sex to distract you from something else you want to be doing

Emotionally detaching from you after sex

Using you for sex, 'booty calls' for example

Ignoring you after sex

Forcing you to do things you are not comfortable with, and then berating you for it (a 'lose-lose' situation)

*

Forcing you to have sex with their friends

Getting their friends to rape you

Having sex with you while you sleep (rape)

Assaulting you while you sleep

Taking humiliating photos of you and using them to threaten or demean you

Bragging about your sexual activity to others

Telling people that you are frigid

Making you beg for sex

Making you feel ashamed or embarrassed for wanting sex

Making passes at your friends

Comparing you to your friends

*

Claiming if you don't give them sex, they will get 'blue balls'

Claiming if you don't give them sex, they will perform badly at work

Threatening to have affairs at work if you don't give them sex

Making you feel insecure, and then laughing or trivialising your feelings

Telling you that you are 'over-sensitive'

Demanding sex **AFTER** you have split up

Telling you that you owe them sex

*

Being overbearing during sex

Threatening to rape you

Tying you up or restraining you when you are not comfortable

Forcing you to say their name over and over

Using household objects to penetrate you during sex, without your consent

Taking you by force, but denying that it is rape because 'you are in a relationship'

I want to give a real-life example of an ex-partner trying to control using sexual contact. We were separated, I did not love him. He was becoming increasingly controlling over my day-to-day life, which had nothing to do with him.

We went to visit my grandmother and grandfather, who was extremely ill. They both knew that we were separated. I was supposed to sleep in the spare room, on a blow-up mattress. My ex-partner was having the double bed. He insisted we share the bed. I said no, I wasn't comfortable sharing a bed with him. He argued with me for over an hour, insisting that as we were technically still married, we had to 'keep up appearances.'

I insisted no, I was not comfortable, and wanted to sleep by myself. He would not have this, using 'God' as a tactic (he was a born-again Christian), also using my grandfather's illness to try and manipulate me, by implying they would both be happier if they saw us 'together.' I said no, they are both aware we are separated, there is no need to lie. Every fibre of my being was physically repulsed at the idea of sharing a bed with this man, I did not want to do it. He was very overbearing, and I was so upset, I nearly gave in.

I'm glad I didn't. I strongly believe that if you are not comfortable sharing a personal or inappropriate space with someone, then you shouldn't have to. I'm glad I didn't give in, that night or any night thereafter.

Earlier that evening, my grandfather had taken me aside and told me, 'Don't do anything you are not comfortable doing.' I was forever grateful for those words.

Another example of sexual control:

I was deeply unhappy, and I didn't want to be in the relationship any longer. He rejected me a lot sexually during the relationship. Towards the very end, when I was falling for someone else, the controller initiated sex which was extremely unusual. He did something he had never done before: he whispered in my ear the entire time, while tears of disgust and revulsion ran down my face. My eyes were squeezed shut because I couldn't bear to look at him.

He told me afterwards that he had deliberately whispered to me so that I couldn't think about the other person while we were having sex. He was controlling my thoughts. The fact I was upset all the way through didn't seem to bother him.

I believe this sex was initiated as form of control – of showing 'ownership' over his property.

More examples of sexual control:

Demanding oral sex whilst refusing to give it

Making you wear something to cover your face or head during sex, to 'dehumanise' you

Not wanting you to move or speak or respond during sex

Not wanting you to have any pleasure

Demanding sex at inappropriate times, to get your attention back on them

Telling you that you have a sex addiction because you need intimacy

Telling other people that you have a sex addiction as a way to shame you

Any kind of public shaming

A real example: After I separated from a controller, and I had confessed to having sex with someone else after months of unhappiness, he became increasingly controlling, emailing me long emails which I would receive at work. These emails were long, aggressive, and abusive, making demands that were unreasonable. As I became harder to control, he then sent out a long, humiliating email to every friend and family member on my contact list, detailing my childhood problems, and that I had a sex addiction, which he was asking everybody to acknowledge and to join him in an 'intervention' for my personal safety.

I remember shaking with shock and adrenaline. Of course, various friends and family responded to him, making it clear how inappropriate and bizarre his email was, and to let me get on with my life. Several forwarded the email to me, as he had sent it without me knowing. I nearly had a breakdown over this email, and I could finally see how frighteningly manipulative and controlling he was when things didn't go his way.

Things to keep in mind:

Sex can be forced or withheld.

Sex by coercion IS a form of rape.

Sexual control has nothing to do with love, and everything to do with power, and having your attention on them.

Further support:

RASAC (Rape & Sexual Abuse Support)

Women's Aid

Domestic and Sexual Abuse helpline – open 24/7 - 0808 802 1414

Email: info@dsahelpline.org

There is also support on the NHS website, as well as on the MIND one.

www.nhs.uk

mind.org.uk

Things you can do:

Keep saying NO.

Log everything that feels abusive in a notebook or on your phone if it is safe to do so.

Talk to a trusted friend or a support group. Make sure somebody knows what is happening to you. Make sure you have somewhere to go if you need to leave.

Talk to Women's Aid.

Build up your physical strength any way you can.

Areas of control…

Emotional

I want to make something clear here; **all** areas and forms of control are emotional. There won't be individual examples in this chapter, but there will be different tactics. All control is emotional because it relies on other people **allowing** the control to happen, and reacting or responding to it in the way that the controller wants, in order for it to work.

A good quote to keep in mind: "Hell is the impossibility of reason."

When you get roped into a controlling relationship, you get caught up in a form of hell that damages you emotionally and health-wise. No wonder; it includes behaviours and tactics designed to make you think you are crazy (gaslighting, denial, isolation, compulsive lying) as well as to demonstrate to others around the controller that you are crazy, thus compounding your isolation.

I have ended up with fibromyalgia and chronic fatigue, as well as blood cancer, and I am no longer surprised to learn that most women I know with these types of chronic illnesses, which can be contributed towards by chronic stress, have a history of toxic relationships (or are still in one).

It is also worth noting that cancer feeds off stress. Stress can literally kill us, and it can stop our bodies and minds from functioning properly. It alters cells, and damages your brain. Not to mention chronic stress is simply awful to experience.

At the height of my abusive relationships, I used to wonder what it would take from me to make the controller happy.

Should I quit my job.

Should I stop having friends.

Should I have plastic surgery to make my figure what he wants it to be.

Should I stop confronting him on anything.

Should I stop asking questions.

Should I try and become a 1950's housewife, stop going out, and convert to Christianity.

Should I stop being me.

But there is nothing. Ultimately, you can shut down every essence of who you are and becoming a walking, talking bot, subservient, never arguing, being who a controller wants you to be, wearing what they want you to wear. But then ironically, you wouldn't be the person that attracted them in the first place; the person full of love and light and empathy, to balance out their lack of. And they STILL wouldn't be happy. Because deep down they are insecure and unhappy. That is **why** they have to control constantly; it is the only way they can deny their shame and feel better about themselves, by putting themselves 'above' someone else.

Nobody happy and full of love ever had to control other people.

Abuse is wrong and abusers know it is wrong. If abuse was really okay, then abusers would just do it, without trying to cover it up. But as it is known to be wrong, it needs to be covert, with many tactics alongside to cover it up, to hide the effects of it, to make it look or seem acceptable, to make us think it is our fault somehow.

One example of controlling behaviour on its own may not seem devastating. But over time, many instances of this equate to a **thousand tiny cuts.** The damage they cause to a person's character and self-esteem is sometimes lifelong.

The complications of control and why it is so hard to define

There is often a huge amount of overlap with control tactics, which makes it even harder to define. I want to give an example of this, to show how a scenario can involve several different types of control:

Your partner doesn't want you to go out, and so they belittle and undermine you until you get upset and therefore don't go out. (This is EMOTIONAL control and attacks your SELF-ESTEEM.)

In the same instance, their belittling and undermining tactics may upset you, but you may still be determined to go. After all, you are looking forward to seeing your friend, whom you haven't seen in ages. You are dressed up ready and looking forward to a catch up. The controller's behaviour may escalate to PHYSICAL control, where they body block you or use their fists to attack you. They might push you or lock the door. Obviously, this would be frightening and bewildering. This would cause you a lot of shock, as well as increased fear for your safety. This PHYSICAL abuse could work and stop you from going out because you are afraid, and don't want to upset the controller further.

The controller could then resort to tears and grovelling apologies in order to force you to stay and feel sorry for them. Your pity and kindness can be manipulated, as they could convince you to stay home and look after them because they know that you are a caring person, and they can manipulate your love for them. This is more EMOTIONAL control.

They may also bring FINANCIAL control to the same scenario. For example, they might hide your purse or your bank card, so that you don't have the means to go out. Or they might claim that you are wasting money. One woman I knew used to have her shoes and her house keys hidden by her controller, so that she couldn't leave the house. He would always deny hiding them of course, and then they would turn up back in her handbag again once the 'rebellion' had calmed down.

The result is the same, you see? Whatever form (or forms) of control worked, whether emotional, physical, self-esteem, they did not want you going out, and they succeeded in stopping you. You didn't go out. You responded and reacted to the tactics and allowed them to affect your plans.

Pathologically controlling people are not capable of ever really caring about your feelings beyond a superficial level; all they care about is winning and getting their way. Their need for control and obedience stems from a deep-seated insecurity that most controllers will never acknowledge or attempt to change. If you are with a controller who is genuinely capable of personal insight and change, then you are one of the lucky ones, because there is hope for a healthy, happy relationship.

Keep this in mind if you find yourself constantly cancelling plans and putting your happiness on hold, to appease the controller. Keep in mind that they can never have enough control over you; nothing will ever be enough. **You can roll over and be passive, trying never to upset them, aiming to give a controller your full constant attention, love, adoration, support – it will never be enough.**

Emotional control covers all means of control really, so I want to shine a light on a few different tactics of control. The controller may favour one or most styles, or they may rotate through them when the early methods fail. Here are some of the few that psychologists and experts have identified:

Gaslighting : this is basically manipulating you into questioning reality. On a basic level it is pathological lying, sometimes to an almost constant degree, and expecting you to believe these lies.

The term 'gaslighting' comes from a 1930's film called Gaslight, where the unscrupulous husband of an emotionally fragile woman aims to drive her mad, so that he can have her committed to an asylum and steal her money. One of the methods used in the film involved the gradual dimming of the gas lights around the house, over a long period of time, and then telling her it was all in her mind, when she started noticed the reduced light.

Gaslighting is extremely insidious, and can involve a variety of tactics including lying within the lie, diverting, being disarming, questioning you, changing the subject, ignoring or 'dismissing' your feelings or thoughts, or acting hurt and confused to confuse you and send you off-track.

It also often involves a 'stuck record' tactic, whereby the controller states the lie in a cool, calm manner, again and again. The lie can be a big thing, but ridiculously, it can be the smallest thing. As much energy goes into getting you to believe the small lies, as it does the big ones.

What matters to them is getting you to give in and believe the lie. They do not care that they are hurting you. They may repeat the lie to others, and over time, you will have heard the lie so many times that even years later, you may find yourself doubting the truth. No presentation of facts or evidence will generally deflect them from their lie; once they are committed to the lie, they won't back down (unless this itself is a tactic to disarm you.)

A couple of examples of bizarre gaslighting, that are still memorable to me many years on:

One of the earliest I remember from my child's father, was after she was born. We were in hospital, and as she was very premature, she was born weighing 4lbs 11 ounces. That number is of course ingrained in my mind, as her mother.

*It was noted down by midwives, written on the tag on her hospital cot, etc. There was ongoing **visible** evidence. Yet her father kept insisting that she weighed a completely **different weight**. He argued with me about it and kept telling the incorrect weight to family who visited, meaning that I had to keep correcting him. Eventually he started to devalue the staff at the hospital, implying that they were neglectful and getting the weight wrong. It was very hard because at the time I was fragile and doubting myself. I even put this weird lie down to him genuinely making a mistake or being forgetful. It was only later that I realised that he was a compulsive liar, and that this lie was one of hundreds.*

Another example of completely pointless gaslighting:

I am a shoe size 5, always have been. The controller bought me some shoes which were the wrong size. He tried to convince me that I was in fact the size he had bought me. I remember arguing, exasperatedly, that I was the size I was, and had always been that size!

When I didn't back down on this, he then tried to convince me that I had told him the wrong size (which I hadn't.)

Many controllers will tell you that all their exes were 'crazy.' This is a common devalue of anyone who found them out and called them out on their behaviour. Be wary of anyone you meet who claims this. If you are gaslit enough, of course it will drive you a little insane. That is the whole purpose of the tactic.

Arguing with a compulsive liar is a waste of time and energy. They will not back down, and they will exhaust you. Even when the lie is pointless, they will lie and lie to convince you that you are wrong.

Gaslighting is destructive and disrespectful, and over time, it can be infuriating at its lowest level, and detrimental to mental health at its worst. It can leave you in a kind of passive, 'wide-open' state where you accept all sorts of mental garbage that is coming your way. It can lead to a place where you stop arguing, stop disagreeing, stop questioning even the most appalling behaviours.

Other tactics include:

Devaluing you as a person, telling you and others that you are 'nuts'

Questioning everything you say or do

Guilt-tripping you (playing the victim, acting upset or hurt, sulking)

Humiliating you

Isolating you

Threats (veiled or obvious, emotional or physical, or both)

Claiming they 'know best'

Micromanaging everything/taking over every aspect of your life

Disregarding you (including ignoring you, dismissing your thoughts or feelings, trivialising you and making you feel small)

Trivialising everything they've ever said and done – by claiming they 'just say stuff,' or they 'can't remember'

Trivialising all of your achievements – sneering at you, saying you got 'lucky' etc

Stonewalling you (refusing to communicate or cooperate)

Areas of control:

Self-esteem

This is a tricky area of control to cover, as you could say that **all** controlling behaviours erode self-esteem and confidence over time. However, I think it is an individual enough area to warrant shining a light on, as self-esteem tends to be a big issue for women especially, who have suffered abuse and control. Having our appearance or intelligence attacked can leave us particularly low.

Therefore, as well as listing examples of abuse, I want to also look at ways of increasing your self-esteem, as increased confidence and belief in yourself will impact most other areas of your life in a good way.

With good self-esteem comes a good, fulfilling life, and decisions that benefit us

When we have low self-esteem, we don't have much love for ourselves, and maybe are lacking in the belief that we deserve happiness and love. We can be more likely to be drawn to destructive partners, and even controlling colleagues and friends. Unfortunately, many controllers seem to have a 'radar' for those who are loving and kind, and thus more susceptible to control, because kind, caring people tend to see the good in people, and give them many chances, despite shocking behaviours.

I want to share some tips on increasing self-esteem. Bear in mind it is a lifelong journey, but it is always worth getting on that path, because each tiny baby step does make a difference to us and how we feel.

Increasing our self-esteem and confidence is something **everyone** can do, whatever age we are, whatever our situation or circumstances. Here we go:

- Start questioning your friendships/relationships with anyone who tells you that you are not good, puts you down or makes you feel inadequate.
- Move towards (emotionally, attention-wise) people who you respect, admire, and who make you feel good or inspire you. This can be anyone: family members, friends, Youtubers who inspire or make you laugh… joining a supportive Facebook

group has led to several real-life friendships for me! Just having accepting people to talk to and connect with, makes the world of difference. Get around people who **lift you up**.

- If you have an aspect (or aspects!) of yourself that you struggle with, or don't feel good about, consider seeking support. It could be online counselling (Betterhelp.com are incredible and match you to a licensed therapist; I have a trusted therapist whom I can go back to for support at any time.) It could be finding a support group or website. It could be a YouTube channel. I can almost guarantee that no matter how lost or isolated you may feel, there will be groups or YouTube channels dealing with it. I, over the course of many years, sought out support for dealing with strong emotions, depression, relationship anxiety, toxic relationships, chronic fatigue, blood cancer, and parenting challenges.
- Listen to an inspirational speaker called Louise Hay. She began to change everything for me, gradually, over time. Her CD/audio recording 'How to love yourself' cannot be underestimated. Listen to it even if you don't believe it. And if you don't want to listen to her, start following her first step, which is…
- Stop. Criticising. Yourself. Just stop it. It may not be easy, but you can begin.
- Get your body moving in some meaningful ways. When we move more, and feel fitter, we hold our head up just a little higher. When we care for our body, we are communicating to ourselves that we value ourselves, and we are also communicating this to the world, to other people. Controllers, like bullies, may 'pick on' those they deem weaker than themselves. Show them who's boss. **Get stronger**.
- Do things **YOU** enjoy. Do some stuff purely because **you** want to.
- Find what makes you laugh or brings you joy; stand-up comedy, gardening, chatting to friends.
- Allow yourself to be human. We all make mistakes; life isn't a perfect straight line. See everything as a brilliant opportunity

to achieve something, to learn, or to grow. Just because we've had several awful relationships, it doesn't mean that we can never experience something better.

Some examples of controlling behaviours relating to self-esteem:

Putting you down

Laughing at you

Calling you names

Insulting you

Criticising you constantly

Disregarding who you are as a person

Disregarding your feelings

Ignoring you

Dismissing your thoughts, feelings or ideas

Making you feel small

Making you feel hopeless

Making you feel that nobody else will love you or tolerate you

Making you feel 'less than'

Making you feel not good enough

Making you feel unintelligent

Criticising your clothing, your style, your hair, your make-up

'Feeding' you so that you stay overweight, or forcing you to eat lots

Taking control of your eating, or of an eating disorder, so that you rely on them and do not seek outside help

Making you feel that your friends or family don't like you

Hiding items and then convincing you that you are 'clumsy,' 'forgetful,' 'useless'

Making you feel like a bad parent

Undermining your parenting decisions

Telling others that you are a bad parent

Undermining your decisions

Taking credit for all decisions and circumstances

Refusing to talk to you when you need help or are upset

Accusing you of 'overreacting' whenever you need to talk about something

Refusing to talk about the relationship

Refusing to acknowledge you as their girlfriend/partner etc

Hiding you/refusing to let you meet their friends and family

Keeping you 'in your place'

Constantly telling you that they are 'too busy' to talk or see you

Not making time for you except on their terms

Only contacting you at night/making you feel like a 'booty call'

Lying to you about their whereabouts or activities

Refusing to see you as a sexual or sensual person

Treating you like a 'mate'

Control types:

Children (AKA: attempting to co-parent with a controller)

I want to add a section about control of children that you may share with a controller, or, just as difficult; an *ex* controller, because aside from my own twelve years' worth of experience (ongoing) plus the dozens of stories I have heard from other survivors, this is not something I see written about, and the standard advice of 'going no contact' and 'running a mile' is just not helpful when you share custody of a child.

Ultimately, you have to find ways to stay sane and cope with the drip-feed of ongoing abuse via your relationship, as well as raising your child as best you can, **plus** managing the knock-on effect of the abuse your child will be experiencing.

I lost count of the number of times people said to me, "Ah well, at least your child's father is around in her life," even after I had talked about the hell that I had been through including court battles, continued lies about my ability as a parent, and the knock-on effects of narcissistic abuse (manipulation and gaslighting) on the child that you love and care for so much. In a strange way, you are still being abused via your child, so even if you have escaped the romantic clutches of this controller, you may still have much more difficulty to navigate around, especially if you co-parent and your child legally lives with both of you.

In our case, our child lives the half the week with me, and half with her father. This arrangement protects not only both parents, but the child's needs too. However much you may despise your ex and what they put you through, a child generally needs both parents. There are exceptions to this; obviously if the child is being severely abused physically, sexually, then they must be removed for their own safety. I tried arguing that emotional abuse was having just as much effect on my daughter; sadly I got nowhere, even when CAFCASS were involved. Controllers can be extremely charming and seem reasonable. Until they slip up, of course.

Things are definitely feeling easier now that my daughter is older, as we have become extremely close, and she feels safe with me. She no longer rages at me because of the influence of her father, and she can talk to me about anything. I am finally able to enjoy the love we share and the fun we have together, and her father is very rarely discussed any more. I think that possibly she understands things a little more, and observes the behaviours and manipulations more than she lets on. One theory is that her father has a new girlfriend, and so she will be the main 'supply' for him now. Also, as our daughter grows into a teenager, she is becoming more independent, and sure of herself as a person. Already she has her own interests, influencers that she follows, plus an open, creative, and good-natured view of the world.

I'm sure her father senses this shift, and maybe doesn't attempt to influence the things he now has less 'say' on.

Trying to seek outside help

Sadly and frustratingly, I have found that there is very little that can be done. I don't wish to detail my daughter's mental health struggles here, but for a few years it was extremely hard to be her parent at times.

I sought help for her mental health via the GP several times, but they would not help due to her young age. I was advised to go private (which I cannot afford.) When I mentioned that her father was narcissistic and abusive, constantly telling her lies about herself and the world, and that I had logged many hundreds of instances, I was advised to 'set up mediation between the three of us.' I was gobsmacked, and of course didn't pursue this. You cannot successfully mediate between a dominator and their victims. They lie constantly, and manipulate doctors, solicitors, the mediation team.

It reminded me of working at a University years ago, where one of the Managers was very controlling and difficult to work with. Picture a female 'David Brent' from 'The Office.' When a young female colleague put in a complaint against her, she cornered her in the ladies' toilets to ask her why she had complained. The girl was intimidated, in tears, and withdrew her complaints. The University, in a twisted attempt to 'calm the waters' decided it would be a good idea to book a meeting and have everybody involved in one room, with this impossible manager. I said no;

it's one of the few times I strongly spoke up against bullying in the workplace. I was just appalled.

I have no idea of the outcome of that meeting. I DO know the young girl had repeated bouts of shingles, and eventually left because of stress. I believe the difficult manager had a nervous breakdown and left or retired. Bullying needs to be faced head on, and not placed on the shoulders of the victim.

*

For the sake of positivity, I shall focus here on what DID ultimately help my daughter (and what is still helping):

Seeking a mentor for my child through a charity (Mentorlink, or some kind of Buddy system).

Seeking additional support for her through her school (most schools have pastoral or sensory support services for children with additional needs or home difficulties).

When she was old enough, getting her a little phone to help her forge bonds with family and friends she could talk to (especially as the controller isolates her and doesn't allow playdates whilst she is with him). The phone REALLY helped, and I saw a big surge in her confidence and sociability.

Having a pen pal.

Going for walks when we got stressed.

Reading stories every night.

Finding relaxation or counselling apps together, so that she can reach out for help on her own terms.

Childline has a really good website, with not only instant chat available with online counsellors, but they have little fun games that help mindfulness and relaxation.

This may sound obvious or go without saying, but it needs to be said, because when you are dealing with crushing stress, constant

triggers and anger at the controller that can't easily be released, it is easy to forget this simple plan for you and your child:

Have fun. Laugh wherever you can. Play board games, watch Disney films, connect, go for walks together or to the park when things get tense in the house and you feel like you might explode.

I used to spend hours talking and TALKING to her with my head in my hands from exhaustion and frustration, going around in circles, especially when I was being blamed for things (an extension of the abuse I got from him, hence very triggering.)

I'd forget how to have fun with her, how to lighten the mood, how to be a mum without a toxic hangover hanging over me day and night.

Get help wherever you can, as you'll need support. Nobody is an island, and nobody can manage everything alone.

Talk to friends, get them involved in your family plans, so that you have as many positive and kind role models around you both as possible. This can help negate the negativity and oppressive atmosphere your child may be suffering with whilst with the controlling parent.

Make your time with them precious, a safe space for them to be themselves, to learn about real love.

For years I felt crippling guilt for 'breaking up our family.' Then I felt guilt that I couldn't stop him manipulating her as he had done me for years. Soon I realised I'm not God, and I can't control everything. What I **can** influence is what happens during **my** time with her. I can teach her love, curiosity, that it's okay to be open and talk about things.

I can teach her about the world, about kindness, about attitudes. In particular, I can model **honesty** by being an honest and open mother. I am showing her how to be healthy. In demonstrating healthy relationships, she can start to see what is **unhealthy**, and question things for herself. I can help her grow and develop and decide what is the best way to live life.

With support for yourself, and the support of partners, friends and family - it CAN be done.

Kindness, honesty and fun are truly in the simple things; you don't need lots of money or specialist equipment to bake cakes or biscuits together, or grow things in the garden, or help out local charities. You don't need a load of high-tech to play a board game together, even Hangman. Get retro, old-school. Go for a walk and look at nature and water; study stuff you find interesting. Take photographs. Meet friends. Just mess about and have fun.

Here is a list of examples of controlling behaviours regarding a child. Some are frequent and ongoing; others appear to be developing as the child hits certain milestones, gets older, etc. It is hard to explain, and obviously I do not get to observe what happens whilst she is with her father. All I observe is her behaviour, her anxieties that can flare up after spending time with him, and also of course; what she tells me (or doesn't tell me).

Almost like a researcher, over the past ten years, I observe the same patterns over and over. By spotting the patterns it helps you detach from it and not take it personally. I can guarantee there will be times you will get stressed, and want to tear your hair out from exasperation. But remember this: The rules haven't changed. Don't react to his provocations or accusations. Don't give him the 'supply' (attention) he craves. The behaviours can change and develop; **the controller's need for control stays the same, no matter the circumstances.**

Examples:

The controller poking their weak spots and teasing the child (to lower self-esteem)

Them disregarding her as a person with her own interests

Focussing on 'results' in order to deserve praise (conditional love)

Putting them down

Pushing them too hard physically

Dressing them in inappropriately (the wrong gender, wrong size, clothing that is similar to their own clothing)

Lying about their care

Refusing to return them to you

Refusing to collect them

Threatening court proceedings if you argue with them or disagree about something

Being secretive about activities

Being secretive about school trips, requirements etc. Withholding necessary information from you

Forcing the child to keep secrets

Sabotaging the child's endeavours

Guilt-tripping the child into sparing their feelings and worrying about upsetting them constantly

Threatening the child that they won't see their parents again if they 'speak up'

Denying that the child has an injury or an illness / lying about what illness

Telling the child to 'man up' when they are hurt or needing comfort

Refusing to accept anything from you during hand-over (clothing, medicine, toys. Strangely this still happens – even carrier bags that have come from my house come back to me, neatly folded)

Telling others that you are negligent (this includes doctors, solicitors, the school, Magistrates)

Fabricating allergies or childhood deformities that don't exist

Creating drama around circumstances so as to cause the child emotional distress or guilt

Constant lying about silly things – I want to show how these petty lies and gaslighting can affect a child's confidence and relationships with their peers:

*My child told me that her and her father had walked 80 miles in a day. I responded that it's simply not possible on foot. I suggested maybe it was 8 miles? 26 miles is a marathon, and that can take 12 hours if you are walking. She argued ferociously that they **had** walked 80 miles, because 'that's what daddy had told her.'*

I knew he was talking rubbish but I had to change the subject as she was getting very upset. When she went to school the following day and told some friends, a couple of them said her dad is lying. Sadly, I think it may have started to click in her head at this point that her dad doesn't always tell the truth. I've had gentle conversations with her about lies, and about how some people lie because they're insecure and want to impress people. I'm trying to focus on kindness, rather than putting her father down.

Using lies about the school as part of an agenda to try and get her home-schooled (by him, surprise surprise).

Refusing to take the child shopping for Mother's day, your birthday etc. This results in huge anxiety for the child (which weakens the child in the controller's eyes)

Trying to get a girlfriend to 'replace' you as a mother.

Devaluing you in front of the child

Phoning the police to report you for 'domestic abuse' because you have confronted them or tried to discuss something

Controlling the child's friendships (in the controller's eyes, people are either 'your' friend or 'his' friend.

Not allowing the child to have playdates without his supervision, even when the child is getting too old for constant supervision

Feeding the child junk food such as three sugary donuts, when they know that you will going on a car journey

Throwing a spanner in the works to try and jeopardize holidays, days out etc

Withholding court orders from the school

Refusing reasonable requests for information

Being belligerent with school teachers and staff

Belittling medical services (even if they themselves initiated use of that service – this tends to happen when they have been neglectful and you have had to take over making appointments i.e. when they have lost control)

An example:

The controller was taking the child to her eye tests but was starting to miss appointments. I informed him that I would sort it, and when he didn't respond, I went ahead. The opticians told me she had missed a few appointments now, and it could impact her eyes, which were getting steadily worse. They told me that she needed to be wearing her glasses all the time, especially at school. I mentioned this to our daughter, who told me that the controller had told her she didn't need her glasses.

I started taking my daughter to her eye appointments. When I mentioned progress and updates to him, I was ignored. Then he started telling our child that 'some opticians were more qualified than others,' and that he knew a 'top' optician in London he would talk to. (It has not happened yet). I did some research, and obviously confirmed that he was lying yet again. All opticians in the UK have the same qualifications. He has now dropped all attempts to take care of her eyes.

Advice for if you are planning to escape

DO NOT TELL YOUR ABUSER THAT YOU ARE PLANNING TO LEAVE, ESPECIALLY IF THEY HAVE BEEN VIOLENT WITH YOU, OR IN THEIR PAST.

Call Refuge – they have a 24-hour Helpline: 0808 2000 247

They also offer online live chat.

They won't tell you what to do, but they will support you and help you make a plan. They can also let you know about local services that can help you, including a refuge if needed.

Some further tips from Refuge (from their website – www.refuge.org.uk)

Create an emergency bag, containing items such as cash, keys, important documents, phone numbers, clothes etc. This could be kept safe with a neighbour or friend, if there is a risk the abuser could find it.

Make a plan. Think about the abuser's routines, when they may be out of the house, so that you can leave safely when he is not home. Plan a route.

Arrange a place to stay, such as with a trusted friend or family member. Or a refuge. Any local authority has to help you if you are a woman fleeing domestic abuse – even if you are not local.

Consider how he might track you i.e. having access to your phone or messages. You may also want to delete your internet history relating to seeking support. You should also turn off any geo-location settings on your phone. Consider using a friend's phone or getting a cheap PAYG phone for private use.

Some further advice:

GOV.UK has information about how to get help with dealing with domestic violence, including how to access help and support, how to spot the signs, and how to get a court order, or a non-molestation order to protect you / your child(ren).

Bright Sky app is a mobile app and website for anyone experiencing domestic abuse, or who is worried about someone else. The app can be downloaded free from app stores. Only download if it is safe to do so.

Women's Aid were a fantastic help for me, when I needed to talk to someone and discuss my options. They even offer group or single therapy sessions (there is a waiting list). They always have fully trained and experienced female support workers available to help.

You can email them: helpline@womensaid.org.uk

They also have an online live chat service, available 7 days a week, from 10am – 6pm.

The live chat can get very busy; but do keep trying. There is also a Survivor's Handbook available on the website, which includes ways to help and support your children.

Other things you can do:

Talk to your employer, or a trusted colleague. Your employer should have access to ways to help and support you if you are not safe in your home, or at risk of stalking by an abuser.

My friend Rie Pearson is the bestselling author of 'Be Kind, No Excuses,' and was a policewoman for over twenty-five years, as well as working with survivors and perpetrators of domestic abuse. I asked her a couple of questions:

1. **What would be the first bit of key advice you would give to a person who was planning to escape from a violent or abusive relationship where control is high?**

Answer:
Plan and have support. This is High Risk time! Speak to Women's Aid.

2. **What are, in your experience as a police officer, the biggest red flags that can indicate serious harm in the future?**
Answer:
There are several high-risk factors:
Separation
Pregnancy/new birth
Isolation
Escalation
Stalking

Rie is keen to add that there is no crystal ball; there really is no way of predicting accurately whether a controller is capable of harming you. That is why it is always safest to leave a relationship early when controlling behaviours are apparent.

What helped others survive and escape

Even during the bleakest times, we can find many small ways of caring for ourselves, of showing ourselves that we do matter, and we do value ourselves, even if someone is abusing us. There are always ways that we can show defiance and fight this, in whatever ways are safe for us to do.

I set up a focus group while finishing off the editing for this book, so that I could not only use my own experiences but could speak to other women who had also experienced and survived toxic relationships. I wanted to have a chapter that focused on the things that helped others survive and stay sane (although how sane we are after a toxic relationship is debateable!)

I was particularly interested in what helped women who ultimately managed to **break free.**

Here are some key things that helped women survive and eventually escape:

Positive / funny / absorbing podcasts

Going to the library

Having a vision board / inspiration board

Rebelling against what the controller wanted, in terms of personal grooming

Eating the food that she wanted to eat, instead of the junk the controller wanted her to eat

Boosting confidence by making friends online in a forum, and in person

Watching TED talks (YouTube) on inspiring subjects, especially listening to women who escaped abusive relationships

Buying a dog, so that the dog could be walked by her and get her out of the house

Enjoying her body physically

Focussing on the children, on the joy they bring

Going running – to bring feelings of freedom and release endorphins ('happy' hormones)

Having friends and family who can gently point out how unhealthy the relationship is, and give support, which ultimately helped this woman escape

Going to her GP – seeking counselling

Giving things time – 'time is a healer'

Having a notebook and logging all the abusive or confusing events. Letting a trusted friend see what is in the book; it can be incredibly validating to have someone else say to you, *"Oh my God – that is not right. Did that really happen to you?"* A log-book can also be vital if you speak to the police at any point

Caring for the controller's dog, taking on all responsibilities. This helped give her confidence, friendship, and the strength to eventually leave because she took the dog with her. It also gave her the strength to fight for a better future

Antidepressants, which helped her feel strong enough to leave

Talking to Women's Aid, who are supportive and will help you come up with a plan

Seeking private counselling

Joining exercise classes

Pursuing creative projects and passions – anything from cultivating a garden, to writing a blog, to knitting scarves

Doing little tasks for yourself, such as getting out for a little walk and posting a letter; this gives you a bit of freedom, a sense of achievement, as well as doing something physical

Using relaxation apps, plus apps for mental health

Reading books on assertiveness and self-help

Getting ANGRY about how you are being treated! Anger can be a great motivator, especially if it is not an emotion you often allow yourself to feel. Channel that anger into activity or action

Retail therapy

Going out with friends

Wanting to be a better role model for daughter

Talking to other mums in a support group

Family members who helped and gave her a place to stay

The charity Safer Places

Focusing on the positive things in life

All coping strategies are valid. Whatever keeps us going and gets us out of that toxic situation.

Strategies for dealing with difficult people

This can be extremely difficult and cause huge amounts of stress. It is important to try and develop the right mindset in order to be able to protect yourself from the insanity of control. Controlling, negative people will try to suck you into their vortex of **doom**, and if you are not careful, you will find yourself susceptible to their controlling tactics once again.

You have to be especially careful in the case of controlling exes, as you may find them turning the charm on you at a later time, if they find themselves single again (or suspect they may soon be). This charm offensive is known as 'hoovering,' and can include telling you that you have always been 'the one,' bombarding you with messages and photos, sending you an 'accidental' text to get your attention, telling your friends that they 'miss you,' fake apologies – whatever tugs at your heartstrings and makes you think about him in a new light. Don't fall for it. It is manipulation designed to get them **SUPPLY** (attention).

Whether the toxic person is the father of your children, a family member, or a difficult friend, here is some advice for staying sane in their presence, as well as practical tactics for dealing with these extremely difficult people.

- Keep in mind that they likely will **never change**. They are not reasonable, self-aware people like you or I. You will have to stop fighting the pointless battle of trying to change or improve them. Get on with your own life and focus on **your** happiness and peace of mind.
- Stop 'feeding' their need for attention. They thrive on your reactions; in fact, they need them. Learn about going 'grey rock,' which is basically giving them very little to no attention or validation. Becoming a very calm, cool, unreactive presence whilst around them. Controllers, specifically narcissistic personality types, thrive on even very negative emotions such as when you argue or get upset or annoyed with them.
Initially, they may work even harder to wind you up, to draw out some kind of emotional reaction or trigger in you. You

have to stand firm and, as Dr Ramani states on her YouTube channel, keep saying to yourself, 'Serene, serene, serene!' Eventually the controller will get bored and 'discard' you, which can be very triggering for you, especially if it reminds you of a neglectful parent. You have to remind yourself that this is what you **want**, and you have to stay strong.

- If you get caught up in conversations with them, **nod and smile**, and seem pleasant. Don't get annoyed or wound up. **Use a mobile phone or a fidget toy** to distract yourself if needed. Excuse yourself and go talk to better, more positive people.
- If difficult people keep offering unwanted unhelpful advice, and are disregarding your boundaries, have a stock answer ready: *"That's interesting advice, I'll keep that in mind."* Then go live your life exactly the way you need to. Some people are oblivious to other people's needs or may lack empathy. Take a deep breath, thank them for the advice, and **move on. Limit your time with this person if you can. Or take moral support with you.**
- Act happy and sociable around exes. Weirdly, the happier and more positive you are around a controller ex, the more it seems to annoy them. They will shut down. They will stonewall you, probably in exactly the same way as when you were in a relationship with them. Be a beaming beacon of light, and **repel** them.
- If you need to, go to the toilet and count to ten. Let out some tension. Text an understanding friend. It can be hard staying calm in front of someone who drives you absolutely mad, but it is important to display a calm energy that has no appeal for them because **they can no longer control you**.
- If you have good news to share, share it with the happy, supportive people in your life first. Only share with the controller or difficult person if you have to. And if you have to, do it **with other people present. Controllers need to look like the good guy in front of others.** The controller will amend their behaviour in front of others, or, if it is too much to bear, they will scarper. Good!

- Another way I find can help deal with an impossible person, particularly an ex-manipulative partner, is to play dumb. Our brains tend to jump quickly to *'Oh, here we go again,'* or immediate annoyance when they start rambling on, attempting to engage us with their lies and manipulations. We can sidestep this a little by saying to them (and to ourselves) *"Oh, how interesting! Oh really?"* And just smiling and nodding, without asking any further questions. By doing this over time, you make it apparent that you will always be polite (infuriating to them as they want to antagonise you, so that they can tell themselves and other people how unreasonable you are). You are also making it apparent that you will **NOT** rise to their bait any longer.
- You can learn to **pity** them. Not to the extent that you get sucked into their lies and mind-games again, or think that you should help or 'fix' them, but because it allows you to not be consumed by irritation or bitterness. Feel sorry for them because they will never have happiness like you will, they will never be able to have relationships without being consumed by jealousy, insecurity and a violent need to control anything. Be grateful you are a healthy person capable of love and the full range of emotions!
- Re-assert your boundaries. It can be hard to not see things in a 'black or white' way, especially if you have very strong emotions around that person. For your own peace of mind, it is perfectly fine to reassess how much time, and what kind of time you want to give to that person.

  With one controlling, negative person, I stopped meeting up with them because they continued to push through boundaries that I had set. They sulked and got in a huff, and offered to end the friendship as they were upsetting me. I didn't react immediately as I didn't want to feed her need for placation.

  I told her I was happy to stay friends. But I also made it clear that meeting up and negativity was not something I had the energy for.

- **Live your life**. Don't give that person too much attention. It's hard, but you have to put your own peace of mind first.

- Find ways to laugh and have fun. Remove yourself from stressful situations where you can.
- Keep going – you **CAN** do it!

Thank you so much for reading this book. I hope it has helped enlighten you, and I hope, if any of the situations were relevant to you, it has helped you begin the journey of **breaking free**.

*Please leave a review and tell a friend. I appreciate it muchly. Keep rocking and being **you**.*

EVA XXX

Printed in Great Britain
by Amazon